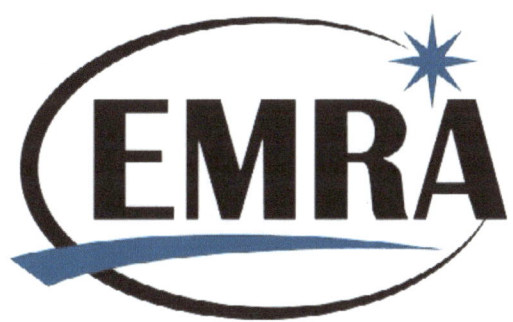

EMRA **Transgender Care Guide**

EDITOR-IN-CHIEF
Christie A. Lech, MD, MHPE
Assistant Program Director
NYU Bellevue Emergency Medicine Residency
Assistant Professor
Ronald O. Perelman Department of Emergency Medicine at NYU Langone Health

CLINICAL INSTRUCTOR
Julia Paris, MD
NYU Bellevue

RESIDENT PHYSICIAN
Aiden Shapiro, MD
NYU Bellevue

EMRA Board of Directors 2018-2019

Omar Maniya, MD, MBA | President
Hannah Hughes, MD, MBA | President-Elect
Zach Jarou, MD | Immediate Past President
Tommy Eales, DO | Secretary/Editor, *EM Resident*
Nathan Vafaie, MD, MBA | Speaker of the Council
Karina Sanchez, MD | Vice-Speaker of the Council
Erik Blutinger, MD, MSc | Resident Representative to ACEP
Sara Paradise, MD | Director of Education
Angela Cai, MD, MBA | Director of Health Policy
Greg Tanquary, DO, MBA | Director of Membership
Nick Salerno, MD | Director of Technology
Eric McDonald, MD | ACGME RC-EM Liaison
Scott Pasichow, MD, MPH | EMRA Representative to AMA
Geoff Comp, DO, FAWM | Ex-Officio Board Member
Sarah Ring | Medical Student Council Chair

EMRA Reviewers

Sara Paradise, MD
EMRA Board Director of Education
Fellow, Multimedia Design Education Technology (MDEdTech)
University of California-Irvine, Department of Emergency Medicine

Erin Karl, MD
EMRA Education Committee Vice Chair of Medical Student Education
Emergency Medicine Resident
University of Nebraska Medical Center, Department of Emergency Medicine

Publisher

Copyright 2018
Emergency Medicine Residents' Association
4950 W. Royal Lane | Irving, TX 75063
972.550.0920 | emra.org

All rights reserved. This book is protected by copyright. No part of this book may be reproduced in any form or by any means without written permission from the copyright owner.

DISCLAIMER

This handbook is intended as a general guide only. While the editors have taken reasonable measures to ensure the accuracy of all information presented herein, the user is encouraged to consult other resources when necessary. The publisher, authors, editors, and sponsoring organizations specifically disclaim any liability for omissions or errors found in this handbook or for appropriate use.

Table of Contents

Introduction 1
(Julia Paris)

Chapter 1. Trans Patient Risk Factors 2
(Julia Paris)

Chapter 2. Terminology 4
(Julia Paris)

Chapter 3. Guide to the History and Physical 6
(Julia Paris)

Chapter 4. Medical Transition 10
(Aiden Shapiro)

Chapter 5. Gender Affirming Surgeries and Complications 12
(Aiden Shapiro)

References 15

Introduction

Transgender, or trans, patients represent a diverse group of people who interact with the health care system and the ED in a variety of ways. Trans patients may be involved with the medical system intensely and for long periods as they align their bodies with their internal identities. In addition, in many cases transgender patients represent a high-risk population with specific care needs.

As transgender health is an emerging field, a large knowledge gap exists among providers when caring for these patients, and this leaves many health care teams inadequately prepared to establish effective communication with their LGBTQ patients, increasing the risk of less-than-optimal care. It's essential for emergency physicians to be aware of the unique approach to care for trans patients.

We hope this guide will help doctors become more familiar with the specific social and care needs of their trans patients, which in turn will help those patients feel more comfortable and encourage them to seek care in the ED.

> **A survey of EM residency programs in the United States showed that only 26% of EM programs had presented a single lecture on LGBTQ health, and only 33% reported some incorporation of LGBTQ health in the curriculum, with an average of 45 minutes spent on LGBTQ content.**

CHAPTER 1

Trans Patient Risk Factors

Much has been done to raise awareness for the health care needs of the Lesbian, Gay, Bisexual, Transgender, and Queer (LGBTQ) community. The National Transgender Discrimination Survey performed by the National LGBTQ Task Force and the National Center for Transgender Equality,

the most extensive survey of trans disparities ever undertaken,[1] details the ways in which trans patients represent a high-risk population. Results showed that, compared to the general population, trans people are 4 times more likely to live in extreme poverty and have double the rate of unemployment. This in turn affects their access to health care, with 4% using the emergency department for primary care. In addition, rates of suicide attempt are 5 times higher than the general population, and the rate of HIV infection is 4 times the national average, with higher rates of illicit drug use, sexual assault, intimate partner violence, and sex work for income or shelter.[1]

Emergency departments serve as safety nets for high-risk patients. Inherent in our training as emergency physicians, we attempt to offer care without bias or prejudice 24 hours a day, 7 days a week, and 365 days a year. Unfortunately, transgender patients frequently report feeling uncomfortable in the ED and, as a result, avoid seeking care for fear of discrimination and embarrassment. One of the largest peer-reviewed research papers exploring ED utilization patterns of trans individuals demonstrated that 21% of trans patients reported avoiding ED care for fear of discrimination.

Another issue was the perceived lack of knowledge on the part of health care providers, with more than half of those surveyed reporting trans-specific negative ED experiences. Similarly, another study found that in cases when inappropriate or disrespectful language was used towards trans patients, providers reported they did not know enough to provide care to these patients, and/or felt ill-equipped to educate other providers about trans issues.[2]

Research has shown a lack of teaching of transgender specific care in medical schools and emergency medicine residency programs. Specifically, in a survey of 132 medical schools in the United States and Canada, only one-third reported teaching about gender transitioning and gender affirmation surgery.[3] In terms of Graduate Medical Education, a survey of EM residency programs in the United States showed that only 26% of EM programs had presented a single lecture on LGBTQ health, and only 33% reported some incorporation of LGBTQ health in the curriculum, with an average of 45 minutes spent on LGBTQ content.[4]

> **Emergency departments serve as safety nets for high-risk patients. Inherent to our duty as emergency physicians, we strive to provide high-quality, sensitive care to all patients 24 hours a day, 7 days a week, 365 days a year.**

Trans Patient Risk Factors

- 4% turn to the ED for primary care

- 21% avoid ED out of fear of discrimination

- 5x more likely to attempt suicide

- HIV infection rate 4x higher than national average

- Higher rates of drug use, sexual assault, domestic violence, and sex work

- 4x more likely to live in extreme poverty

- 2x more likely to be unemployed

> **One of the largest peer-reviewed research papers exploring ED utilization patterns of trans individuals demonstrated that 21% of trans patients reported avoiding ED care for fear of discrimination.**

CHAPTER 2

Terminology

One of the most important aspects of the doctor-patient interaction is establishing a rapport and making patients feel safe. Research has shown that poor patient–provider communication is strongly associated with adverse health outcomes.[5]

When caring for trans patients, understanding and utilizing correct terminology is the initial step in establishing effective communication, making patients feel comfortable and welcome in the ED.

But gender terminology and identity is quite complex; for example, Facebook has more than 50 different gender options, and the list is constantly expanding.

Sex refers to the biological and physiological characteristics that define men and women.

Gender refers to socially constructed roles, behaviors, activities, and attributes society considers appropriate for men vs. women.

What is *transgender*?
When a person's internal sense of gender identity or expression does not align with their sex assigned at birth

What is *transsexual*?
When a person alters their body via hormones and/or surgeries to align with their sense of gender identity. *This term has largely fallen out of favor.*

What is *cisgender*?
A person whose current gender aligns with their birth sex

What is *gender nonconforming*?
A person whose appearance and behavior do not conform to societal expectations or cultural norms of what is appropriate for each gender

What is *gender fluid*?
A person who does not identify with a fixed gender identity, and their sense of gender may fall somewhere on the spectrum between male and female, as well as change over time

What is *gender non-binary*?
A person who does not choose to identify as male or female or feels their gender is outside the binary of male or female

What is *trans*?
This is a term often used to describe the entire trans, non-binary, and gender non-conforming community

What is *AFAB* or *AMAB*?
This term stands for Assigned Female At Birth/Assigned Male At Birth and can be used to describe people who fall in a variety of current gender categories but have a particular birth gender

What is *TGNB*?
This stands for Transgender/Non-Binary and is a term used to include various people whose gender does not match that assigned to them at birth

LGBTQ

This acronym is often changing, and various letters are included in different permutations. In this resource we are referring to Lesbian, Gay, Bisexual, Trans, and Queer people. However, in other settings you might see Questioning, Intersex, Asexual, Allies, or Two Spirit people included specifically.

Examples
1. **Transgender male/man:** a person who is born female sex, but their sense of gender is male
2. **Transgender female/woman:** a person who is born male sex, but their sense of gender is female

This is by no means an exhaustive list, and the language surrounding gender identities is rapidly changing every day, and from place to place. A person's sense of gender is not always binary as in "male" and "female" and may fall somewhere on the spectrum between the two or may change over time.

Pronouns

While general terminology helps familiarize the provider with the trans/non-binary community, the most important terms to establish with a patient are the pronouns the individual prefers.

While some may prefer the gender-based "he/him/himself" or "she/her/herself," there are many other variations. Others may prefer more gender-neutral pronouns, such as "they/them/themselves" or "ze/hir/hirs/hirself" or "ze/zir/zirs/zirself." While these are some of the more common pronouns, there are many other examples. It is best to simply ask the patient what pronouns they prefer.

> **"In a situation where your patient's gender may not be apparent, it is best to simply ask them what pronouns they prefer."**

CHAPTER 3
Guide to the History and Physical

Presenting to an ED can be anxiety-provoking for all patients, but especially so for trans patients. It is critically important to create a safe, sensitive, and trusting environment by employing specific questions, terminology, and physical exam techniques.

The first rule: Do not make assumptions! Specifically, do not assume a patient's gender, sex, or sexual orientation until clarifying with the patient.

This chapter will review how to establish a rapport with trans patients, and provide specific history-related questions and terminology to use when asking these sensitive questions. An overview of physical exam approach and techniques will also be reviewed, with specific regard to patients undergoing hormone therapy and in the setting of gender-affirmation surgery.

History
Name + Pronouns
Start by establishing by what name and pronouns the patient would like to use, as this may differ from what is recorded in the chart. Simply ask, **"What name and pronouns do you prefer?"** Getting this right is the single most important thing you can do to put trans patients at ease.

If you make a mistake with language, be sure to apologize prior to moving on. Patients will appreciate your recognition of the error.

Sex + Gender
Explore the patient's sex and gender identity, as these are two distinct entities for the transgender patient. *Sex* refers to the biological and physiological characteristics that define men and women, while *gender* refers to socially constructed roles, behaviors, activities, and attributes society considers appropriate for men vs. women. Keeping questions open-ended is extremely important, as it gives the patient an opportunity to describe themselves in their own words. For example, ask **"What sex were you assigned at birth?"** or **"How would you describe your gender identity?"**

Hormone Therapy + Gender Affirmation Surgery
Not all trans patients will be taking exogenous hormones or will have undergone surgical approaches to alter their physical appearance. Thus, it is important to obtain this history from every trans patient in order to provide appropriate care. An easy initial question to broach this topic is, **"Have you pursued any changes in your appearance or body to bring it closer to your sense of self?"** If the answer does not elicit specific information about hormone and surgical history, then probe further. Ask **"Have you ever or are you currently taking exogenous hormones or any other medications related to gender presentation?"** If the answer is yes, be sure to ask where they are getting these hormones, as some patients may be taking unregulated hormones they buy online without the guidance of a physician.

With regard to surgical history ask, **"Have you ever had or thought about having any surgeries to align your body with your gender?"** Knowing if your patient has had surgery, and what kind, will help guide the physical exam.

It is also important to ask patients about tucking, which may be done by transgender female patients who have not undergone gender affirming surgery. It is performed by manually displacing the testes upward into the inguinal canal, and then positioning the penis and scrotal skin between the legs and rearward. Applying tight underwear, tape, or a gaff (special garment) helps to maintain this positioning. Prolonged periods of tucking, which places the urethral meatus close to the anus, may result in urinary reflux or infection, such as epididymo-orchitis, prostatitis, or cystitis.

Some trans men who have not undergone top surgery may bind their chests, and if this is done too tightly or for an extended period of time, it can put these patients at risk for rib fractures, atelectasis, or even pneumonia.

Sexual History

Transgender patients have higher rates of engagement in sex work and HIV infection. Because of this, every physician must take a detailed sexual history in order to tailor their care appropriately.

Start with the familiar, **"Are you currently sexually active?"** but also obtain specific information as to what kind of sex (oral, anal, and/or vaginal) and with whom (men, women, both, other). For example, a transgender male may still have female reproductive organs, and if they've had vaginal receptive intercourse with a cisgender man, they need to be screened for pregnancy. They are also still at risk for diseases such as ovarian torsion and pelvic inflammatory disease. Additionally, this patient may need referral to a gynecologist for regular check-ups, including pap smears. It is important to approach these questions with particular detail to language, and ask patients what kind of language they use to refer to their body. For instance, some patients may be uncomfortable with the term "vagina" and may use another term instead. In addition, a transgender female may have male reproductive organs and is at risk for diseases such as prostatitis, prostate cancer, and testicular torsion. In general when taking a sexual history, it is always a good idea to ask about the pelvic organs your patient has, as well as those of their partners, and once again try not to make assumptions.

Social History

Transgender patients are at a higher risk for intimate partner violence, suicide, illicit drug and alcohol use, and homelessness, when compared to the general population. Screening for these entities is a key part of the history, and referral to social work is important so patients know what resources are available to them.

Approaching the topic of violence can be uncomfortable, but it cannot be avoided. Initiate the conversation by asking, **"Have you experienced physical, sexual, or emotional violence recently?"**

All patients should be screened for depression and possible suicidality. Providers can use the Patient Health Questionnaire-2 (PHQ-2) to screen for depression. Ask, "**How has your mood been? Have you been feeling depressed or hopeless? Have you ever thought you would be better off dead? Have you thought about hurting yourself in any way?**"

Homelessness is a complex issue for transgender patients - not only because they exhibit high rates of homelessness, but also because finding a safe shelter can be very difficult. Based on where you practice, there may be specific resources and shelter for trans patients, and social workers can help with information and referral.

With regard to questioning about illicit drug and alcohol use, approach this is in a similar manner as you do with all patients.

Physical Exam

This section will provide special considerations to make your trans patients feel more comfortable during the physical exam. First and foremost, do not perform any unnecessary physical exam maneuvers that are not relevant to the patient's chief complaint or invite unnecessary team members into the room, as many trans patients have described feeling like a "specimen" or "spectacle" on display. If you must examine a sensitive area, be sure to ask permission and also explain why it would impact their medical care, as you would with any patient.

Transgender Male

The pelvic exam may be a traumatic and anxiety-inducing procedure for trans men, especially if they have not undergone gender affirming surgery. Again, you can start by asking a patient how they refer to their anatomy and if they are comfortable using words like vagina to describe their anatomy. If a patient has not had gender affirming surgery and thus still has female reproductive organs, but is taking exogenous testosterone, this can induce a hypo-estrogen state, which promotes atrophy, increases vaginal pH, and increases the risk of vaginitis and cervicitis. In order to perform a pelvic exam, it is advisable to use the smallest speculum available, or even an anoscope, to reduce pain and trauma. Give the patient an overview of how you will perform the exam, and alert them of each step before you do it.

Transgender Female

Whether or not a transgender female patient has undergone gender affirming surgery will dictate how you perform the physical exam. For patients who have undergone surgery with vaginoplasty, the recommendation is to use an anoscope for the pelvic exam. After inserting the anoscope, the trocar is removed, and the walls of the neo-vagina can be visualized.

For patients who have not undergone gender affirming surgery, approach the genitourinary exam with sensitivity by explaining everything before it is performed, and pay particular attention to whether a patient practices prolonged tucking.

When appropriate, based on the patient's chief complaint, do not forget that these patients, regardless of surgical history, likely still have a prostate and may need a prostate exam.

TABLE 1. Key History Questions

What name and pronouns do you prefer?
What sex were you assigned at birth?
How would you describe your gender identity?
Have you pursued any changes in your appearance or body to bring it closer to your sense of self?
Have you ever or are you currently taking exogenous hormones, or any other medications related to gender presentation?
Have you ever had or thought about having any surgeries to align your body with your gender?
Have you experienced physical, sexual, or emotional violence recently?

TABLE 2. Key Physical Exam Notes

Transgender Female	Tucking	Concern for urinary reflux/infections (epididymo-orchitis, prostatitis, cystitis)
	Genitourinary Exam	• Use an anoscope for patients who have undergone surgery with vaginoplasty • Take extra care to explain each step, especially for patients who have not undergone surgery
	Prostate Exam	Do not forget your patient may need a prostate exam
Transgender Male	Binding	Concern for rib fractures, atelectasis, pneumonia
	Genitourinary Exam	Use smallest speculum possible, with adequate lubrication
	Pregnancy Test	Do not forget your patient may need a pregnancy test

CHAPTER 4

Medical Transition

Many transgender men and women take hormonal medications to help align their body with their identities. For trans women this mostly consists of estrogen and anti-androgens. These medications lead to many changes in the body such as stopping facial hair growth, body fat redistribution, breast development, and even lactation in some cases. In trans men, this is usually just testosterone, which conversely leads to body and facial hair growth, increased muscle mass, fat redistribution into more male patterns, and clitoral enlargement. While many trans individuals welcome these changes, different people have different ideas about how masculine or feminine their bodies should look, so they may take different amounts of hormones to best align their bodies with how they feel. Some effects of these medications can be more stressful for patients; for instance estrogen can lead to decreased erectile function, while testosterone can lead to hair loss. In addition, these medications typically require a prescription, and depending on state regulations, patients may need a written letter from a mental health professional to begin hormone therapy.

While medical transition is often more attainable for patients than surgery because of cost, it can still be difficult to get access to licensed providers, and some of your patients may get hormones from black market providers, online, or internationally. Some may even use other non-traditional chemicals to alter their hormones in other ways. The most important things to remember are that hormonal changes happen gradually over months to years, some are reversible in varying degrees, and different patients may feel positively or negatively about the resulting changes to their body.

Feminizing Medications

Estrogen

Estrogen is the most common feminizing medication that your female identifying trans patients may be taking. As with cisgender women, venous thromboembolus (VTE) is one of the more common complications of exogenous estrogen use.[6] Again, as in cisgendered women, this risk is further increased in smokers, patients over the age of 40, those with prolonged immobilization or sedentary lifestyles, the obese, and those with underlying thrombophilic disorders.[6] Most women use injectable steroids, although some may prefer pills, patches, or creams. The rate of VTE is decreased with transdermal estrogen.[6] However, many trans women report that feminizing effects happen more slowly with transdermal estrogen, so it is not as popular. There is data to support the idea that estrogen may increase the risk of cardiovascular disease in patients over 50 with underlying risk factors.[7]

Anti-androgens

Most trans women take anti-androgens in addition to estrogen. These drugs reduce endogenous testosterone levels and activity, which then decreases the dose of estrogen needed to suppress the effects of testosterone on the feminizing body, as well as help with a more feminine body fat distribution.[8] The most common of these is spironolactone, which can cause diuresis and hyperkalemia, as well as the development of high prolactin levels and even prolactinoma.[9]

Many trans women also take finasteride or dutasteride, 5-alpha reductase inhibitors that decrease the peripheral conversion of testosterone to DHT, which is the hormone that often contributes to body hair and male pattern baldness.[8]

Progesterone

Progesterone is a controversial medication in the transfeminine community. Some trans women report that it increases energy, libido, and improves breast development and body fat redistribution.[10] However, there is very little data to support those claims. In addition, progesterone may further increase the risk of blood clots.

Masculinizing Hormones

Most trans men only take testosterone, as no medication is needed to suppress estrogen production in order to see masculinizing effects. This is usually taken as an injectable intramuscular shot, although some trans men prefer to use patches or creams.[8] Although there is limited data, some anecdotal evidence does suggest that masculinizing effects take longer with transdermal testosterone.[8] There are limited side effects of testosterone, but there is an increased risk of polycythemia vera, as well as increased LDL and triglyceride levels. Most trans men on testosterone will not ovulate and therefore not have a menstrual cycle, making pregnancy impossible. However, if dosing has been irregular or lower than necessary to suppress this cycle, ovulation and pregnancy are possible. Thus, it is important to rule out pregnancy in all of your patients with ovaries.

TABLE 3. Key Medical Transition Notes

Feminizing Hormones	**Estrogen**	Some increased risk for DVT/PE
	Anti-Androgens	Hyperkalemia, prolactinoma
	Progesterone	DVT/PE
Masculinizing Hormones	**Testosterone**	Polycythema vera, hyperlipidemia
	Genitourinary Exam	Clitoral enlargement, vaginal dryness
	Pregnancy Test	Rule out pregnancy in all patients who could be ovulating

CHAPTER 5

Gender Affirming Surgeries and Complications

While some trans and non-binary people transition their gender socially without changing their bodies, or with only hormone therapy, many choose to have surgery to help align their body with their sense of identity, and to decrease dysphoria. Some of these procedures are small, and fall into the category of minor plastic surgery, while others are more comparable to major invasive surgeries. It is important to remember that there is no one way to be trans or non-binary, and different patients will have had some, all, or none of these procedures. In addition, there is no fixed order in which these procedures must be done, and indeed, many trans people choose never to have some of these procedures. What is important to understand is that there is no such thing as a "complete" transgender person, and your patients' identity is not necessarily tied to their current bodies or genitals, or their plans to change them.

Feminizing Procedures

"Bottom surgery"

Some trans women experience dysphoria surrounding their genitalia and wish to have their penis removed. This is usually done with several procedures including a penectomy, orchiectomy, vaginoplasty, clitoroplasty, and vulvoplasty; typically collectively referred to as "bottom surgery." The basic technique for this involves inversion of the penile skin, placement of a pedicled colosigmoid transplant, and free skin grafts to make up a neovagina. The neovaginal vault is created between the rectum and the urethra, using the penile skin to line the vagina. Labia are created using scrotal skin, the testes are removed, and a clitoris is created from a portion of the glans. Often, prior to the procedure, trans women undergo electrolysis of the penile and scrotal skin to create hair-free tissue.[11] Post operatively, gauze packing or stents are placed inside of the newly created vaginal vault to create a negative space. After the packing is removed 5-7 days later, the patient is usually instructed on the use of vaginal dilators to increase diameter of the neovagina post operatively.

Complications of this procedure include typical surgical complications, such as bleeding or infection, as well as complete or partial necrosis of the vagina, clitoris, or labia if the blood supply is interrupted. This anatomy is also susceptible to bladder or bowel fistulas into the vagina, urethral stenosis, as well as a lifetime increased risk of UTI, as the urethra is now considerably shorter similar to cisgendered women.

Breast Augmentation

Many trans women develop breast tissue if they are taking estrogen and testosterone blockers, and many are satisfied with the appearance of their chest after 12-18 months.[11] However, some women also choose to get breast implants as well to increase their breast size. This carries the risks of any other breast augmentation surgery, such as infection, bleeding, or rupture. In addition, trans women that have had breast implants are less likely to be able to breastfeed, should they desire to do so.

Facial Feminization

Many trans women undergo some type of plastic surgery to create a more feminine facial appearance. This can include alterations to the jaw, chin, cheeks, forehead, nose, and eyelids, as well as hair implants or adjusting the hairline.[11] For some, these procedures decrease dysphoria and allow trans women to be safely present in settings where their trans status might otherwise put them in harm's way.[11]

Tracheal Shave

Some trans women have this procedure done to decrease the size of the thyroid cartilage or "adams apple." A small incision is made under the chin to reduce scarring, and the cartilage is reduced and resized.[11]

Silicone Free Injection

Many surgical procedures for trans people are very expensive, and many people in the trans community have limited access to insurance or health care. In contrast, silicone free injections are up to 90% cheaper than traditional surgery, so they are an appealing option for face, hip, and chest contouring for many people.[11] However, this is not an FDA approved use of silicone, and it carries a high risk of complications. In addition, many people that get free injections do so from non-physician providers, including on the black market, where the silicone may be injected in extremely high doses or contaminated with other substances.[11] These injections can cause infection, necrosis, migration of silicone, allergic reaction, silicone pulmonary embolism, and other organ damage.[11] These complications can evolve over time, or happen immediately after injection.

Masculinizing Procedures

"Mansculpture"

Some trans men feel a sense of dysphoria about their hips, thighs, stomach, or other areas and wish to get liposuction to create a more masculine body contour. Complications are similar to any other liposuction treatment, and include bruising, pain, bleeding, and infection.

Hysterectomy

Many trans men opt to get a hysterectomy, typically with a bilateral salpingo-oophorectomy. In previous decades, this was often a criteria for starting on hormones, as there was some thought that testosterone might increase cancer risk, although this is not supported by current data. Today, some trans men still opt to have the surgery because of a continued sense of caution over possibly increased cancer risk, or dysphoria over having a uterus. Other trans men may wish to keep their uterus and preserve the option of getting pregnant.

Phalloplasty

This refers to the creation of a penis with a free flap or pedicle flap of skin from the arm or thigh, which is then rolled into a tube structure and grafted onto the inguinal area. Typically, the clitoris forms the base of this structure in order to retain erotic sensation.[11] A urethral extension is made from a cheek or vaginal mucosa donor site, and often an erectile implant is placed within the phallus. Complications of this include urinary tract stenosis, loss of erotic sensation, necrosis or infection of the phallus, and wound breakdown, which often occurs at the perineal-scrotal junction. There is also a concern for rectal injury.

Scrotoplasty

Here a scrotum is typically created with skin flaps from the labia majora and testicular implants are placed inside. Often small expanders will be placed within the tissue and gradually filled with increasing amounts of saline in order to encourage new skin growth prior to the surgery and permanent implants being placed.[11]

Metoidioplasty

This procedure allows for the growth of the clitoris, which occurs with long term testosterone injection, to create a small 1-3 inch phallus. After sufficient growth, the clitorus/phallus is freed from ligamentous attachments to the labia and body, with some labial skin further attached to increase girth.[11] Often the urethra is lengthened at this time as well to allow for urination through the phallus. This is called a "urethral hookup" and typically uses skin from either the mouth or labia majora.[11] Some trans men choose to get a vaginectomy or scrotoplasty with this procedure, but it is not required.[11] However, penetration, pap smears, and vaginal exams may be impossible afterwards due to the decreased size of the vaginal opening, if it remains.[11]

Mastectomy

This is the most common procedure for transmasculine people. It differs from other types of mastectomy in that there is more male chest contouring, and most procedures allow for nipple retention. There are several methods of "top surgery", depending on the size of the breasts, skin elasticity, and other factors. The most common is "double incision," where an incision is made above the nipple line, fatty tissue and gland is removed, and then the nipple is replaced above the incision.[11] For smaller breasts, there is also the option of "periareolar" incision, where an incision is made around the areola, and fat and gland are extracted from there, after which the nipple is reattached.[11] Both of these procedures typically require drain placement, often in the axilla. Complications are similar to other types of mastectomy, such as wound infection, drain blockage, or dehiscence. Some trans men and non-binary people with very little breast tissue may opt for liposuction alone, although they should be warned that if they become pregnant this may make their breast tissue more prominent.[11]

REFERENCES

1. James SE, Herman JL, Rankin S, Keisling M, Mottet L, Anafi M. The Report of the 20015 U.S. Transgender Survey. Washington, DC: National Center for Transgender Equality.

2. Bauer GR, Scheim AI, Deutsch MB, Massarella C. Reported emergency department avoidance, use, and experiences of transgender persons in Ontario, Canada: results from a respondent-driven sampling survey. *Ann Emerg Med*. 2014;63(6):713–720.e.1.

3. Obedin-Maliver J, Goldsmith ES, Stewart L, et al. Lesbian, gay, bisexual, and transgender-related content in undergraduate medical education. *JAMA*. 2011;306(9):971–977.

4. Moll J, Krieger P, Moreno-Walton L, et al. The prevalence of lesbian, gay, bisexual, and transgender health education and training in emergency medicine residency programs: what do we know? *Acad Emerg Med*. 2014;21(5):608–611.

5. Stewart M, Brown JB, Donner A, McWhinney IR, Oates J, Weston WW, Jordan J. The impact of patient-centered care on outcomes. *J Fam Pract* .2000;49(9):796–804.

6. Goodman MP. Are all estrogens created equal? A review of oral vs. transdermal therapy. *J Womens Health (Larchmt)*. 2012;21(2):161-169.

7. Maraka S, Singh Ospina N, Rodriguez-Gutierrez R, Davidge-Pitts CJ, Nippoldt TB, Prokop LJ, Murad MH. Sex steroids and cardiovascular outcomes in transgender individuals: a systematic review and meta-analysis. *J Clin Endocrinol Metab*. 2017;102(11):3914-3923.

8. Deutsch M. Medical Transition. In: Erickson-Schroth L, ed. Trans Bodies, Trans Selves: A Resource for the Transgender Community. New York, NY: Oxford University Press; 2014:241-264.

9. Sover Y, Sharon N, YAron M, Yacobi Bach M, Yaish I, Stern N, Greenman Y. High Prolactin Levels in Transsexual Women are Related to the Anti-Androgen Treatment Modality. *Endocrine Society's 96th Annual Meeting and Expo*. June 21-24, 2014.

10. Deutsch M. Information on Estrogen Hormone Therapy. UCSF Transgender Care Website.

11. Chyten-Brennan J. Surgical Transition. In: Erickson-Schroth L, ed. Trans Bodies, Trans Selves: A Resource for the Transgender Community. New York, NY: Oxford University Press; 2014:265-290.

NOTES

NOTES

NOTES

NOTES

NOTES

EMERGENCY MEDICINE BOOKS FOR YOU

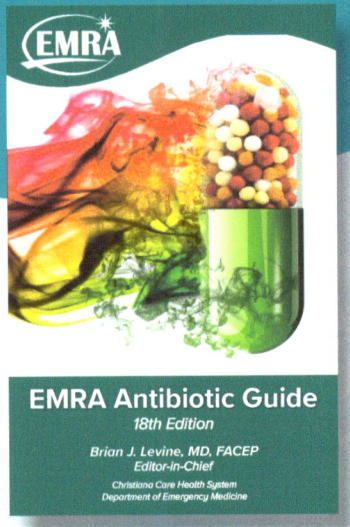
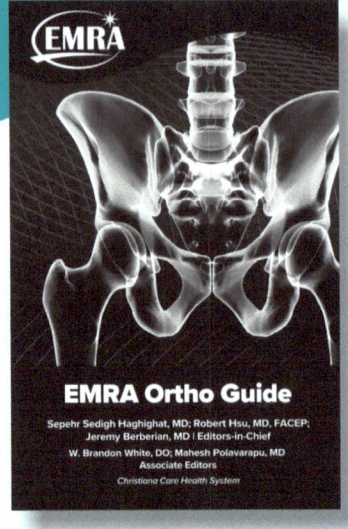
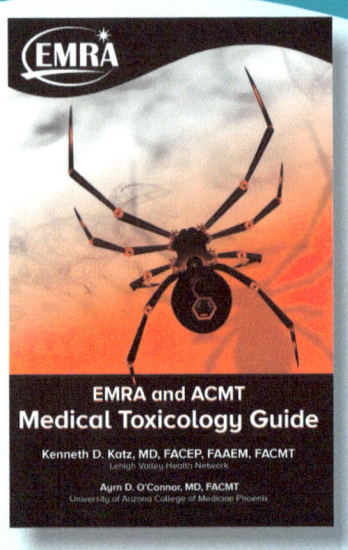
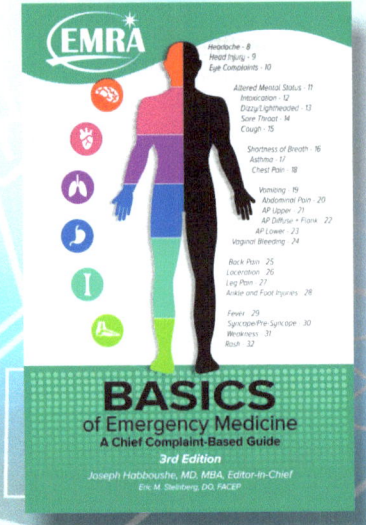
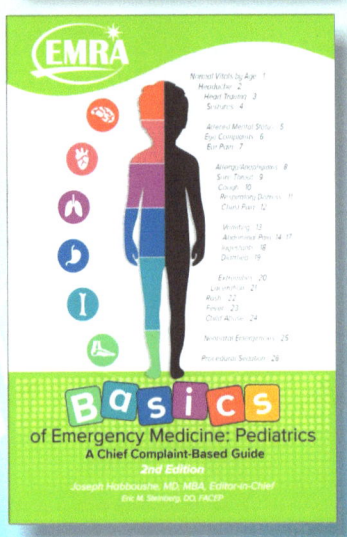
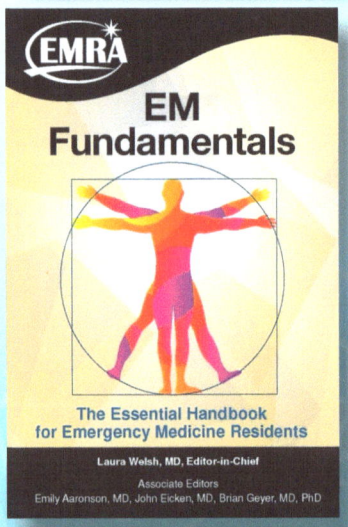
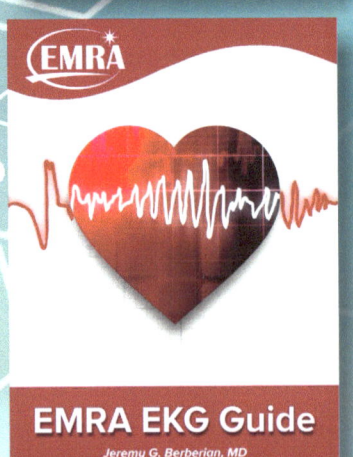
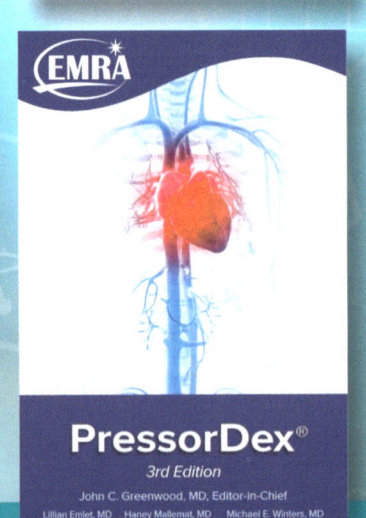
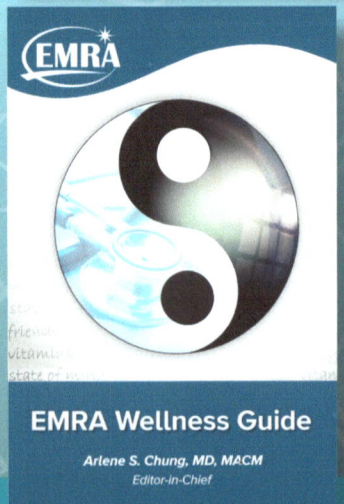

emra.org/guides

www.ingramcontent.com/pod-product-compliance
Lightning Source LLC
Chambersburg PA
CBHW051837210526
45473CB00005B/1912